I0435292

Nicholas G. Stangarone

The GYROCISOR Power Shuttle: Enter The Force Dimension.

Gold Mind Press

All Rights Reserved
Copyright © 2014 by Nicholas G. Stangarone
No part of this book may be reproduced or transmitted
in any form or by any means, electronic or mechanical,
including photocopying, recording, or by any information
storage and retrieval system without permission in
writing from the author.

ISBN-10: 1495217140
ISBN-13: 978-1495217142

Printed in the United States of America

Second Printing

This book is dedicated to the Great Almighty.
The most generous force of all.

Table Of Contents

Chapter One

Muscle Fiber: The Biology of Force

Those aggregate muscle fibers forming our calves, thighs, buttocks, upper arms, shoulders and back constitutes the greatest capacity to generate maximum blood flow while simultaneously displacing the largest volume of respiratory air flow. The author of "Exercise RX," Gary Yanker and his team of medical experts have identified five major muscle-group "movements" capable of producing maximum circulatory stimulation throughout the muscles of the entire body.

Specifically, these five muscle movements are the stepping movement for calves and shins. Then proceeding ever so upwards, we encounter the kicking action for thighs and buttock muscles.

Then moving upward again, we have rotating the torso for the abdominal and lower back muscles. After that, there is the rowing or swimming movements for the arms, chest and upper back. Finally, there's the movement of raising both arms in a continuous fashion.

Just by exercising these five muscle groups results in a vigorous distribution of blood to all of the body's aggregate muscle components and vital organs. The health and fitness benefits from engaging these muscle groups in a strenuous manner are numerous and range from improving overall strength and cardio to promoting balance and coordination.

But more importantly, it also explains why the GYROCISOR Power Shuttle and corresponding "SuperStroke" maneuver become so effective together as a complete health and performance enhancing exercise.

Basically, the Gyrocisor "SuperStroke" maneuver engages the majority of our core muscles in a highly coordinated, bi-lateral elliptical movement that can be performed for any duration that is necessary to attain the desired fitness level. When this movement is combined with the angular momentum of a live and loaded GYROCISOR Power Shuttle, the efficacy of the exercise is multiplied by a factor that is proportional to the speed or additional weight.

But before elaborating further on any particular details describing the GYROCISOR Power Shuttle and "SuperStroke" maneuver, I suggest we attempt to gain a true historical perspective ascertaining the evolutionary trajectory of physical fitness exercise. This should provide the groundwork to fully appreciate how prominent the GYROCISOR work out will stand in the pantheon of effective exercises.

Let's first begin by admitting to ourselves while cozily reclining on a pillow clad overstuffed couch, that without a doubt, the truly arduous nature of scrambling to survive the ice age was a daily workout. Especially, with only the most rudimentary means of hunting and fishing, life demanded exhaustive feats of physical strength and stamina. Arguably, the force of this ancient struggle has to some extent, etched itself onto our genetic code. And possibly, this ancient genetic mutation is made clearly evident by our body's proclivity to react beneficially to reasonable amounts of strenuous physical exertion. And it could be said by simple observation, that human beings not only require adequate shelter and a well-balanced diet to maintain health and fitness, but also physical activity. Especially in the form of exercise denominated activity.

One of the earliest depictions of ancients exerting themselves in exercise has been dated all the way back to the distant reign of the Egyptian Pharaoh's, nearly four and a half thousand years ago. It's clearly a remarkable rendering in that it seems to portray the lifting of heavy objects for no other discernable purpose than as would be required for weight resistance training.

Particularly curious is how this small group of ancient Egyptian bodybuilders appear engaged in the act of swinging clubs that are very similar to those used by the fearsome warriors of India when they were trained for battle. And so it would seem that after thousands of years and the emergence of the British Empire as a global power without peer, one of the spoils of conquest was the archaic practice of swinging heavy clubs for improving overall physical fitness.

And this is important because it must have been shortly after the very first pair of Indian clubs arrived on the shores of the English Isle that similar implements began percolating across the short hop over the channel to the European mainland.

Consequently, by the middle of the nineteenth century or in other words, nearly 5,000 years after those hieroglyphs depicting Egyptians exercising with clubs, a similar pair of those clubs invaded the fertile shores of America with the initial waves of hardy immigrants from the German provinces.

As previously mention with respect to the quantity of strenuous exertions that had been constantly demanded of man's early prehistoric adaptation. It would also stand to reason that any form of military combat prior to the introduction of gunpowder should have demanded a similar amount of highly intense physical activity.

Personally, I believe that the introduction of chemical explosives cuts a sharp line of delineation that demonstrates how technological advancements have so effectively diminished the relevant nature of man's powerful muscle momentum while engaged in the heat of battle.

So it's rather ironic that one of the earliest examples of military fitness comes from the Chinese Chou Dynasty, way back during the tenth century BC. Since, of course, gunpowder made its way into western hands by way of the eastern brain. Yet, it's there that the conscription of military recruits first required they perform specific feats of strength just to qualify for enlistment.

Another example of ancient physical fitness was the martial predicament of young Spartans. Upon reaching the age of seven, the youngsters were torn from their mother's comforting care. Then they were rudely subjected to the most strenuous ideals of a military nation-state. For the next twelve years of their formative lives, these hardy youths were forcibly extruded into those exemplary warriors of eternal legendary acclaim.

And the men charged with forging these tender buds into hardened Spartan soldiers were called the Paidonomos. Dreaded taskmasters and obvious forerunner of today's drill instructor, many of these men surely delighted in drilling the young Spartans beyond the merciless boundaries of fatigue and fear. Yet, these cute, pintsize warriors did grow to manhood. A body of men, who were able to endure the toil of hunger, thirst and cold, even as they constantly trained for battle with little or no sleep.

While this torturous form of physical fitness was accepted within the realm of their societal norms and taboos and hardly possible in our indulgent lifestyles. It also stands as irrefutable proof that strenuous activity or exercise exists as a genetic component of our evolutionary endowment. In other words, human muscle fiber not only responds favorably to strenuous exertion; muscle hungers for force to thrive and grow strong.

It's also worth considering that as early as 776 BC, man's endowment of strength, speed and agility was famously celebrated during the first Olympiad. And though that inaugural Olympic Game had commenced with a foot race. Surely all those in attendance would have revered Hercules with the same esteem afforded their other powerful Gods residing atop Mount Olympus.

But whether the feats of Hercules were fact or fancy, one cannot doubt the voracity of that Macedonian prince. The young and gifted general, who conquered the Persian Empire with the unmistaken skill of military genius.

But why was Alexander the Great followed over half the known world? Was it because of the genuine fraternal affection, he had shared with his men. Or perhaps, his courageous willingness to head their invincible battle formations. Maybe it was, though less dramatically, Alexander's endearing eagerness to forego daily affairs of state and exercise alongside the ordinary infantryman.

And it's not by sheer coincidence that the principles of progressive resistance made famous by Milo of Crotona to attain superhuman strength are still valid to this day. For as legend states, Milo had built his strength by gradually increasing the "weight resistance" over a considerable period of time. That is, by simply lifting a young calf onto his back at least once a day until the animal had fully grown, his muscles were able to adapt to the increased weight. Pretty rudimentary, but it still forms the bedrock for strength training and muscle building routines, twenty-five hundred years later.

Another ancient who also impacts modern life is Galen, that preeminent physician from the Ancient Roman Empire. As doctor to the Legions, Galen not only developed surgical techniques still used today, but he also found time to prescribe a series of training exercises for fitness training. Of particular interest, some of his exercise routines also included the use of halters. The legitimate precursor to the modern dumbbell because they were used for the specific purpose of building athletic speed and strength.

Obviously, looking good at the baths while chit-chatting with the locals of ancient Rome was just as important then as it is to look hot at the beach today. We know this because of the ample room provided at the most Roman baths for those who wanted to work up a sweat pumping some weights. Fortunately for Caesar, he didn't need to wear a muscular cuirass to sport a sexy six-pack.

When time came for the classical world to fade into the shadows of barbarism, the necessity for daily exercise was replaced by extreme physical hardship. And unfortunately, this highly strenuous condition would persist in one form or another for several centuries.

Not surprisingly, it would take the cultural and intellectual clarity that swept across Europe as a contagion from the Italian peninsula to finally escape the opaque reasoning of the Dark Ages. For it was the European Renaissance that rekindled the classical desire to build muscular physiques according to the long lost exercise routines of their ancestral fitness enthusiasts.

And within a century or so, well give or take a decade, anyway sometime during the middle of the sixteenth century, numerous accounts of freakish human strength suddenly began to appear. Was this an indication of the increased curiosity such feats of strength could stir up among the common gentry?

Certainly, something was beginning to stimulate demand in building muscle growth and power through "progressive resistance" exercise. Perhaps, it's partially attributable to those traveling carnivals of the Middle Ages and their popular "Strongman" act.

Interestingly, this quest for super human strength appears to have always been matched by a proportional affinity toward a more leisurely or sedentary lifestyle.

And so with bittersweet irony, it would appear that as quickly as we've acquired the technological means to relegate menial and repetitive labor or heavy lifting to mechanical work, we've sought the path of least resistance to the nearest cozy couch.

Unfortunately, this human tendency of aversion to strenuous exertion or heavy lifting can quickly atrophy the average man's muscular physique, making them appear soft and effeminate.

But soon enough, proper attention was directed to this modern, "flabby man" syndrome and people began to seek the means or exercise routines to maintain a strong and vigorous body. So, with "deja vu all over again," the expertise and knowledge of the classical Greco-Roman world to build muscular physiques was back in vogue.

But the dawn of the eighteenth century soon placed those amazing feats of strength under scientific scrutiny. One such incident occurred when the English strongman, Thomas Topham performed his popular "Herculean acts" before the distinguished and highly discerning gaze of the British Royal Society.

Without venturing far off course, It's amazing to think that since the likes of Isaac Newton, this scientific society had diligently investigated the mechanics of gravitational force with the mathematical savvy of his calculus equations. And that their elevated gaze should turn from contemplating gravity's play on planetary motion to the meager capacity of human muscle to generate lifting power. That is, the ability to move a heavy stone against the force of earth's gravity.

So, after Mr. Topham's demonstration of bodily strength before that distinguished body of learned men, a publication was circulated entitled, "Encyclopedia of Bodily Exercises." It effect was to quite literally, spark a physical fitness revolution throughout known Germany. And within a brief period, the "cult of the body beautiful" was soon celebrated across that country with numerous festivals. Some of these served to popularize the use of both the horizontal and parallel bars in many of their gymnasiums.

By 1772, a few years before Hessian mercenaries were disembarking on American shores to manhandle the revolting colonialists under the command of their imperial paymaster, the benefits of exercise were clearly understood by at least one true American patriot.

I find it quite revealing, that is, when one considers how someone like Benjamin Franklin, a middle aged man with profoundly more pressing issues concerning a "state under siege" to occupy his thoughts and time, then to make the effort to write his lumpy, disloyal "Loyalist" son and extoll the healthy virtues of breaking a sweat while exercising with dumbbells.

But whatever may have been the elder Statesman's motivation, another half century would pass unnoticed before an unknown German immigrant started what would become America's first gymnasium in the colonial state of Massachusetts.

And within a generation or two, a rather enterprising physician from that very same state had made his way onto the fitness landscape of that period. It seems that this Doctor Windship hoped to persuade the public that "main strength" or the power to lift heavy weights was simply unattainable by the calisthenics of the nineteenth century gymnasium.

Story has it, that prior to America's Civil War, the good Doctor Windship had braved the unpaved roads of the backwoods frontier to preach his beliefs on the gainful virtues of pumping iron.

And it is by his own accounts that Windship may have been the original ninety-eight-pound weakling. Supposedly, he would boldly proclaim that if even he, once a mere pip squeak,

could acquire such impressive strength, then surely anyone could! But of course, they had to follow his prescribed exercise routine utilizing weights. Not sure if he was selling the weights or just the printed routines. But certainly no DVDs! That would take another hundred and fifty years or so.

But even after such a prophetic venture, it would not be until the 1893 Chicago Exposition, before the musclebound strongman flexed his way to international fame and fortune. But of course, this would be no ordinary strongman that could jumpstart the muscle mania. It would require the skills of a master showman with strong, bulging muscles. It would require the incomparable Eugene Sandow.

Sandow was undoubtedly one of the first to profit from this increased enthusiasm for the spectacle pleasure of flexing, bulging muscles. Because soon after the Chicago Expo, he partnered up with the famous Ziegfeld, who just happened to be an even bigger showman. And before long this master strongman was performing in exhibitions and earning upwards of about thirty-five hundred dollars per week. Quite the chunk of change for a turn of the century bodybuilder.

But more significantly, at least to the muscle world, happened during one of those Sandow performances, when one young spectator was so transfixed by this "Herculean" spectacle, that he would subsequently publish the first fitness magazine in the United States.

By 1926, Macfadden's muscle magazine boasted a respectable circulation of nearly half a million readers. But that notable achievement would not be the sole feather in his entrepreneurial bonnet. Because even before that phenomenal feat, his bounding ambitions propelled him toward producing a series of contests dedicated to finding America's most perfectly sculpted man.

Then, with only a fist full of years into the twentieth century, these fledgling precursors to today's bodybuilding contests were popular enough to be staged at the most legendary sports venue in the world, Madison Square Garden.

However, the full significance of these early "muscle meets" would not be realized until the winner of the eighteenth such event decided to change his name because it was too ethnic sounding. And so became the legendary Charles Atlas and also one of the first successful attempts to mass-market muscle making. Using his masterful publicity campaign, Angelo Siciliano introduced the American public to the unbearable plight of the puny, sand-dusted ninety-eight pound weaklings trembling on beaches everywhere. Suddenly, tender weaklings everywhere had reason for hope in a world dominated by muscle headed bullies. No doubt, the revival of the "scrawny weakling syndrome" would have made Dr. Windship quite proud, up there on muscle beach heaven. A place where all good fitness pioneers like Jack Lalane and many others may probably dwell.

The increased popularity of building muscle or strength that remained in the wake of Sandow, Macfadden and Siciliano was an impetus for the advent of the amateur weightlifter. As this enthusiasm for amateur weightlifting eventually culminated with the 1898 World Weightlifting Championships.

And within less than five years later, the Milo Barbell Company was forged together by a Mr. Alan Calvert to fill the rapidly growing demand for weightlifting equipment. Obviously providing the necessary iron to form a sturdy foundation for what we now recognize as Power and Olympic Weightlifting.

By the time the nineteen twenties were in full roar, the formation of the American Continental Weightlifters Association along with the consolidation of other smaller organizations had crystallized into the AAU or Amateur Athletic Union. But, the impetus for this regulatory body had been set in motion with the introduction of weightlifting at the 1920 Olympic Games. And therefore, somewhat symbolically, the circle that had begun so long ago in the classical world of ancient Greece, two and half millennia earlier, was effectively closed.

The 20th century is credited with the promise of a new world order, but it also brought the brutal realities of two world wars that forced a majority of able bodied men to become physically conditioned for combat or perish. But now, this intense physical exertion would provide all the results necessary to associate strenuous activity with health inducing and recuperative properties. And this on a certain level, takes us right back to Galen and his fitness exercises for the Roman Empire's combative Legions.

Along a similar vein, sometime following World War II, a Dr. DeLorme has been credited with coining the term that's become synonymous for building strength and muscle through the systematic lifting of progressive weight increases.

And though the phrase, "progressive resistance" may have first been spoken during the twentieth century, they would have been thoroughly understood by Milo and his growing calf. So many, many centuries before that it speaks volumes of how the fitness industry has evolved.

Interestingly enough, it's about this same period that many athletic coaches assumed weightlifting was not suitable for enhancing sports performance. Their primary concern was that the athlete would lose too much speed and coordination to perform their sport. But a far worse consequence was that the athlete would become muscle bound. Personally I can also remember that even as late as the seventies, as a high school athlete, I also heard the same cautious advice.

But soon that was to change. And one determining factor was offered by the safety and convenience of lifting resistance on a "Universal Gym" weight training system. Little by little, the lingering doubts faded and progressive resistance machines began to occupy gyms throughout the fifties. Not long after, weightlifting was well on its way to becoming part of every sports performance training regimen.

Yet, the universal gym was not the first exercise machine in America. Even as early as 1740, a rather strange, if not titillating exercise contraption called a "chamber horse" was in use by hopefully just a few early fitness enthusiasts. Supposedly, it was intended to simulate the action of a riding horse. Though, it's probably fair to say, not at full gallop.

The 1870's not only saw the rise of the cowboy gunslinger, but also the use of treadmills. Though not for today's stationary walkers because it was designed to be used for harnessing animal power on the working farm. But it would not be until the 1950's when John Wayne cowboy westerns were all the rage that the first medical treadmill was built to exercise humans.

And while the stationary bike may have been around for as long as the bicycle, the elliptical version would not be in use until 1995. But by then the science of physical fitness was

becoming firmly established as an authentic curriculum at numerous colleges and universities.

One powerful incentive for all the advanced degrees was the amazing commercial success of televised professional sports. This demand for legions of trainers and strength coaches to keep a winning or losing team's expensive talent at peak performance each season has yet to reach its worldwide potential.

And finally as the past decade of the 21st century has ushered in an increasing multitude of exercise routines including "Muscle Confusion" theory, "Hip Hop Abs," Yoga, Pilates and cross-fit training. And to some degree, the "wii" virtual sports, Fitbit and the vast array of sports and fitness apps have certainly added excitement to physical fitness. And of course the ubiquitous nature of YouTube and similar sites along with the mass acceptance of social media has only increased the possibilities of exercise on an infinite scale.

But from a personal perspective from someone who has been following the latest fads and trends in exercise and physical fitness since 1970, the most notable seismic shift in fitness occurred with the complete domination that women now enjoy in the global fitness community. Perhaps it was ushered in by Jane Fonda's Fitness videos from the eighties or just a reflection of the increased participation rate of women in sports or a slew of other reasons combined. Either way, women have created an industry all their own.

Although this was a very condensed version of the historical facts, hopefully you have found it comprehensive enough to delineate a discernable trajectory of the pursuit of physical fitness to our present day. Because a truly dynamic approach to

strength and cardio exercise has arrived to usher in a new dimension in physical fitness; the force dimension.

The ONE alternative strategy to constantly fighting the force of gravity. Because performing the GYROCISOR "SuperStroke" maneuver with a live and loaded Power Shuttle is more like surfing the force of gravity to the star-planet; Hard Muscle. Then, let's say, struggling against Earth's gravity like a bowling ball with butterfly wings.

But that's exactly why, the GYROCISOR make exercise fun; force fitness fun. And over the next few successive chapters of this booklet, all the details necessary to use and build a GYROCISOR Power Shuttle will be presented for your enjoyment. In the meantime, we'll end this chapter with the discovery and development of the GYROCISOR Power Shuttle and the "SuperStroke" maneuver.

First of all, the discovery of the GYROCISOR Power Shuttle and the "SuperStroke" maneuver was a purely serendipitous event. Basically, while in the process of moving cross country with no inkling or desire to invent the GYROCISOR. And as such, lacking any preconceived notion, the significance of the discovery was not immediately evident. And were it not for a personal tragedy, the discovery would never have been fully realized.

In any event, my earliest recollections of the muscle enhancing effects that I've termed, "Quantum Dynamic Tension (QDT) happens in the late summer of 2002. But due to a number of pressing circumstances, it wasn't until February 2004 that the first GYROCISOR Power Shuttle was built. Then over the weeks that followed, I perfected the GYROCISOR "SuperStroke" technique or maneuver. By May of 2004, a demonstration of the GYROCISOR technique using the first GYROCISOR Power Shuttle was videotaped at Del Puerto Canyon in Northern California.

In 2007, after three years of exercising with the GYROCISOR, a very limited attempt to test market under the StangoBango Enterprises (SBE) brand. Within eighteen months, the US economy had collapsed into the Great Recession and all funding suddenly evaporated for SBE.

It was decided to shutter the business, but continue R&D on the GYROCISOR Power Shuttle. Since then, numerous tests have been conducted to determine the exercise stress limits of the GYROCISOR "SuperStroke" technique. These results will be presented in the follow-up publication. Also included in the publication will be the results of the first GYROCISOR GAMES.

This booklet was first published in commemoration of the tenth anniversary of the 2004 GYROCISOR model. This second edition is being released as part of a renewed effort to share the benefits of the best exercise in the universe with all the world.

Chapter Two

The GYROCISOR SuperStroke: Three Exercises Packed In One.

Progressive resistance exercises operate specifically on counteracting the force of gravity or some other alternative form of resistance. By focusing maximum tension to a specific muscle component, it's a highly effective method for bodybuilding and or building strength. The effects of progressive resistance training have been known and utilized since antiquity.

But as important, the bio-mechanical structure of the human body has evolved for 360-degree rotational motion because we exist in a three dimensional world. Constricting this fluid rotation to repetitive linear movement should result in mental and muscle boredom because it lacks the stimulation of full range motion. Eventually this "dumb" movement will squelch the willpower necessary to succeed because of muscle boredom.

And it's this boredom that the GYROCISOR Power Shuttle and the "SuperStroke" maneuver eliminates because the fluid oscillation of the exercise engages every facet of the body in that universal interplay between angular momentum and gravity.

By fusing the movements of chopping wood or axe swing with the rowing exercise and the freestyle swim stroke into one continuous super movement and then combining it with a dynamic "progressive resistance" device like a live and loaded GYROCISOR Power Shuttle, you get the muscle power of Quantum Dynamic Tension or QDT.

Basically what this means is that by compressing these strengths into one comprehensive workout means that this exercise can provide the same physical exertion for the upper body as running does for the lower body minus the jarring impacts with the road surface.

In addition, there are certain similarities to the functional training benefits provided by working the medicine ball. This is because, like the medicine ball, the individual must use his or her core muscles to stabilize their torso for the proper execution of the GYROCISOR "SuperStroke" maneuver with a live and loaded GYROCISOR Power Shuttle.

Also this phenomenal exercise for building core muscle groups incorporates a number of health inducing movements that are experienced in performing Tai Chi. Of course, the primary difference is that the GYROCISOR is loaded with weight and that means you've got the potential for some serious kinetic energy. And that power boost or lift to charge the "SuperStroke" called Quantum Dynamic Tension or QDT is the power you feel throughout the exercise routine. It's all about Newton's third law, you see.

"For Every Action, There's an Opposite & Equal Reaction."

Until now, our focus has centered on the biomechanical aspects of the GYROCISOR "SuperStroke" maneuver. However, another aspect of this space age exercise that delineates itself from other progressive resistance exercises is that the force one experiences with the GYROCISOR is angular momentum and torque. While on the other hand, the type of force generated by the linear displacement of the weight in a typical progressive resistant exercise is the displacement of the weight's inertia and momentum.

It's this alternative force utilization to the exercise that I've termed Quantum Dynamic Tension or QDT. This basically means that when an individual (Gyronaut) is engaged in the GYROCISOR "SuperStroke" maneuver with a live GYROCISOR Power Shuttle, there are additional forces at play besides gravity. These two other force components that are added to the power mix are angular momentum and torque. The results are an incredibly vigorous full body motion within a relatively minimal amount of time and space constraint.

Further, according to Newton's second and third laws, angular momentum is conserved. That is to say, repetitive weightlifting routines like the bench press or squat result in substantial force expenditure to reverse the weight's direction and its momentum. This momentum is basically lost once the weights come to rest in its own inertia.

In stark contrast, during the performance of the GYROCISOR "SuperStroke" maneuver, the angular momentum of the live and loaded GYROCISOR Power Shuttle is never lost because it simply revolves into the opposing direction.

That is, when fully engaged in the "SuperStroke" with a Power Shuttle, the universal force of gravity is longer your tormenting enemy. You know, that unrelenting force that ultimately breaks you down and humiliates to the point of giving up and just quitting like some punk ass bitch.

Instead, when you resonate with the fully loaded, the force of gravity becomes your best surfing buddy. That dude you know, who will always watch your back. Your best friend forever. You don't need to fight gravity anymore because with the GYROCISOR "SuperStroke" maneuver and the Power Shuttle, gravity will work for you. Doing everything it can to help you achieve ever new heights of glorious health and fitness!

The Physics of Quantum Dynamic Tension

The parallels between linear motion and rotational motion can be easier understood and appreciated when compared alongside each other:

Linear Motion	*Rotational Motion*
Velocity – v	w – Angular Velocity
Acceleration - a	a – Angular acceleration
Mass (linear inertia) – m	Moment of inertia $\{I = \frac{1}{2} M(R)(R)\}$
Momentum – (p = mv)	(L = Iw) – Angular momentum
Kinetic energy – $\{1/2 \, m \, (v)(v)\}$	$\{1/2 \, I \, (w)(w)\}$ – Kinetic energy
Force = ma	Torque = m(r)(r)a

The similarities are striking, however rotational motion has one other force component that linear motion lacks and that is torque.

$$\textbf{Torque (t) = Ia}$$

And torque is a leveraged force. The magnitude of the torque (t) of the force (F) about the axis is defined to be the product of the magnitude of the force and the lever arm.

Torque (t) = FD (lever arm D)

This force used to steer or deflect the rotational motion. And since for every force there is an opposite but equal force, you are also privy to this dynamic quantity when you exercise with a live and loaded GYROCISOR Power Shuttle.

Also another advantage of exercising with the GYROCISOR "SuperStroke" maneuver and loaded Power Shuttle can be understood by looking closely at the equation that expresses the dynamic quantity of rotational motion.

K = ½ I (w)(w)

This formula involves the angular quantities, Moment of Inertia (I) and Angular Velocity. The squaring of the Angular Velocity (w) component clearly demonstrates why speed is an influential component of the GYROCISOR "SuperStroke" maneuver.

When the Angular Velocity (w) is squared, the force you put in as speed is doubled! For example, if you double the speed of the "SuperStroke", it will feel as though the force of the weight has quadrupled. That twenty pounds of iron strapped to your GYROCISOR will feel like you're moving eighty pounds of mass!

Of course, that would require that the size of the elliptical orbit remains the same size. When someone is performing a large orbital "SuperStroke," the speed can be increased by tightening up on the orbit or widen out the trajectory to slow it down.

Another more familiar way to consider this phenomenon is to recall the image of the graceful skater exploiting the conservation law of angular momentum by decreasing the distance of her arms and legs from the axis of rotation to induce a faster spin.

Another advantage of the GYROCISOR "SuperStroke" maneuver is that the entire movement can be mathematically described with the analysis of simple harmonic motion. To best image this, we need only think of children playing on a swing. Acting like giant pendulums, they quickly learned to increase the swing by anticipating the best height from which to extend their legs and increasingly forcing a higher trajectory. And that is what it means to resonate with a live and fully loaded GYROCISOR Power Shuttle, you will find that everyone has their own natural harmonic resonance. But each one, no matter how different will always be in true harmonic resonance with the Universe.

And in chapter five, we will learn more of what it means to "Become one with the Universe" and the "Force" will be with you.

Chapter Three

How to Perform the GYROCISOR "SuperStroke" Maneuver.

The GYROCISOR "SuperStroke" maneuver is a highly effective exercise because it fuses together the freestyle swim stroke, the long axe swing and the rowing stroke into one continuous "SuperStroke" movement. When you engage in the GYROCISOR "SuperStroke" maneuver with a live and loaded GYROCISOR, it's like surfing the waves of gravity for an exhilarating way to exercise. The GYROCISOR "SuperStroke" maneuver is a bi-lateral, dual elliptical maneuver that can be repeated in a continuous and flowing fashion.

Of course, in addition to performing the GYROCISOR "SuperStroke" maneuver (infinity movement) and depending on the weight of the live GYROCISOR Power Shuttle, extreme centrifugal and torque forces can be encountered. If you've skipped the previous chapter, you may want to briefly consider that the angular momentum you will generate is equal to the "moment of inertia" multiplied by the angular velocity of the live and loaded GYROCISOR Power Shuttle. So depending on a combination of weight and speed, you could have a loaded weapon on your hands.

So it is of the gravest importance that you begin slowly and with careful attention to the weight you add to the GYROCISOR Power Shuttle. Avoidance of injury at this stage is crucial! Therefore, you should always start off with the lowest weight to induce QDT, if any additional weight at all. That is, until you've mastered the GYROCISOR "SuperStroke" maneuver. Typically, 5 to 10 pounds of added weight to the GYROCISOR Power Shuttle should be safe enough to begin learning to master exercise.

Though the GYROCISOR "SuperStroke" maneuver is performed in an infinite motion trajectory, it can basically be broken down into six distinct movements that starts from the power stance position.

1.) The Power Stance
2.) Quantum Launch Lift
3.) Torque Tilt Drop
4.) The A-Orbital Trajectory
5.) Reverse Torque
6.) The B-Orbital Trajectory

1.) *The Power Stance.*

When engaged in the GYROCISOR "SuperStroke" maneuver the loaded GYROCISOR Power Shuttle can produce severe momentum swings, so it is important to begin in the proper Power Stance. The Power Stance gives you the flexibility, support and control to handle the forces generated by the "SuperStroke" infinity movement.

A. Sound footing is critical. Begin with your feet spaced at least on foot apart and firmly planted. Knees should be slightly bent and with some bounce.
B. Shoulders should be square and parallel to firmly planted foot stance.
C. With back straight, lean slightly forward.
D. With arms extended, letting the GYROCISOR Power Shuttle hang freely.

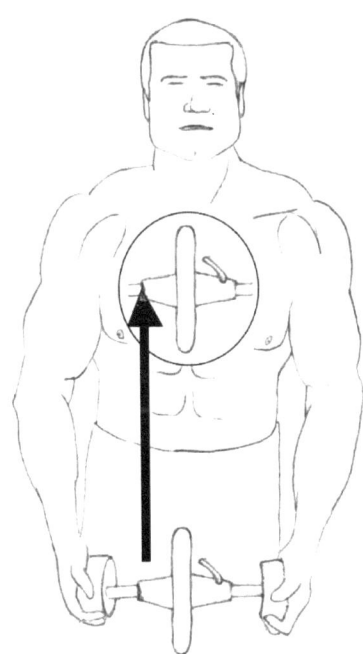

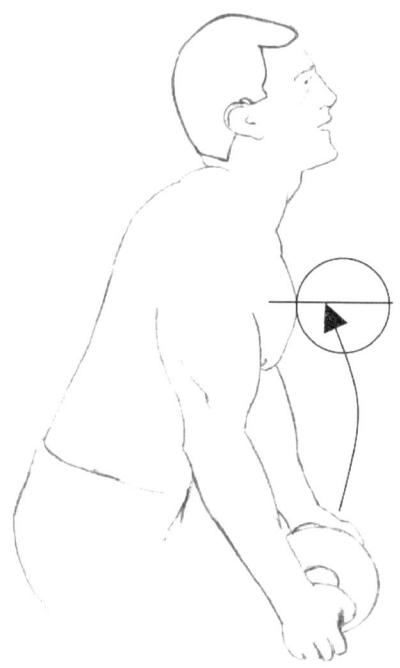

2.) *The Quantum Launch lift*

From the Power Stance, you can safely resonate the GYROCISOR "SuperStroke" maneuver by energizing the loaded GYROCISOR Power Shuttle. To energize a loaded GYROCISOR Power Shuttle, you need to lift it to the required height of potential energy. The force required to lift the GYROCISOR Power Shuttle equals the "Quantum" in the QDT (Quantum Dynamic Tension). The proper height is typically chest high or higher.

Because of the conservation laws previously mentioned, the force you commit to energize the loaded GYROCISOR will remain throughout the entire exercise routine. It is the potential energy that's converted to kinetic energy as you resonate doing the GYROCISOR "SuperStroke" maneuver.

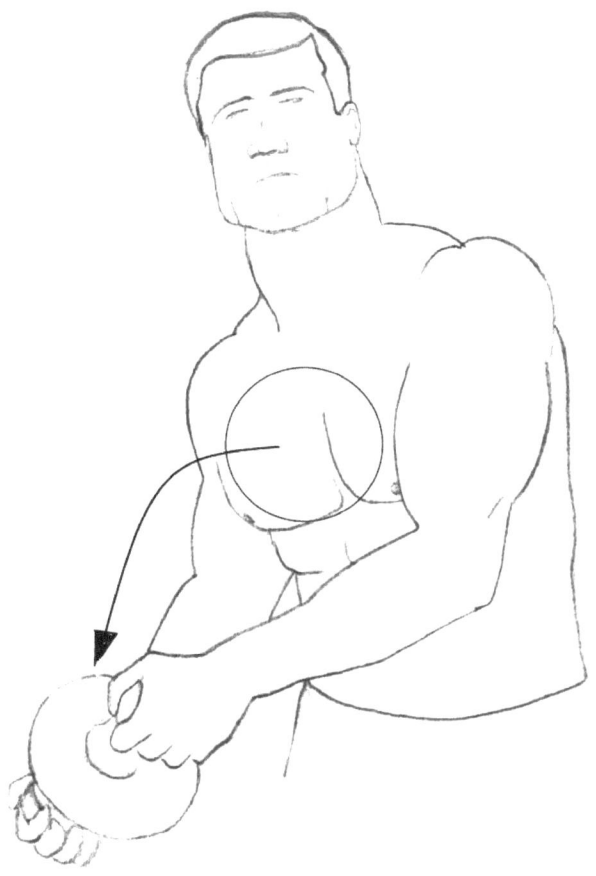

3.) *The "Torque Tilt" Drop*

From the maximum height of the Quantum launch, torque the lead end of the GYROCISOR Power Shuttle down to let it descend into the downward trajectory of the first elliptical orbit. While holding firmly to both grips of the GYROCISOR Power Shuttle allow it to travel in naturally parabolic descent and gain momentum.

For maximum effect, you should bend knees as the GYROCISOR Power Shuttle descends to its lowest point.

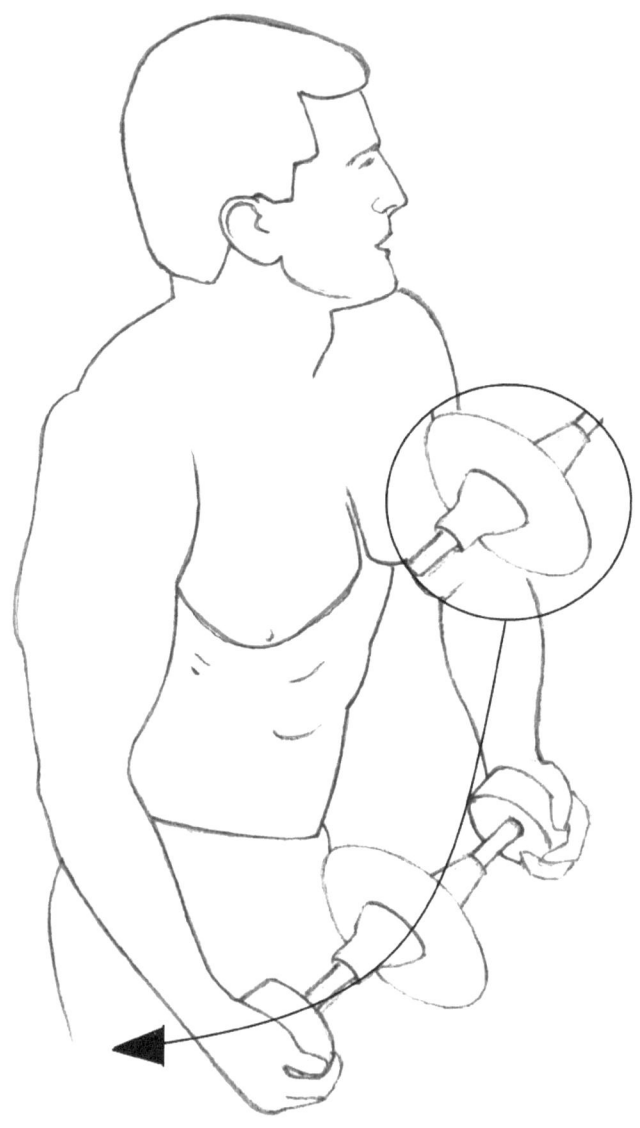

4.) *The A-Orbital Trajectory*

Using the gained angular momentum of the speedy GYROCISOR Power Shuttle to lift the load above shoulder height in flowing elliptical trajectory.

Twist torso and extend bended knees to maximize the height of raised GYROCISOR Power Shuttle.

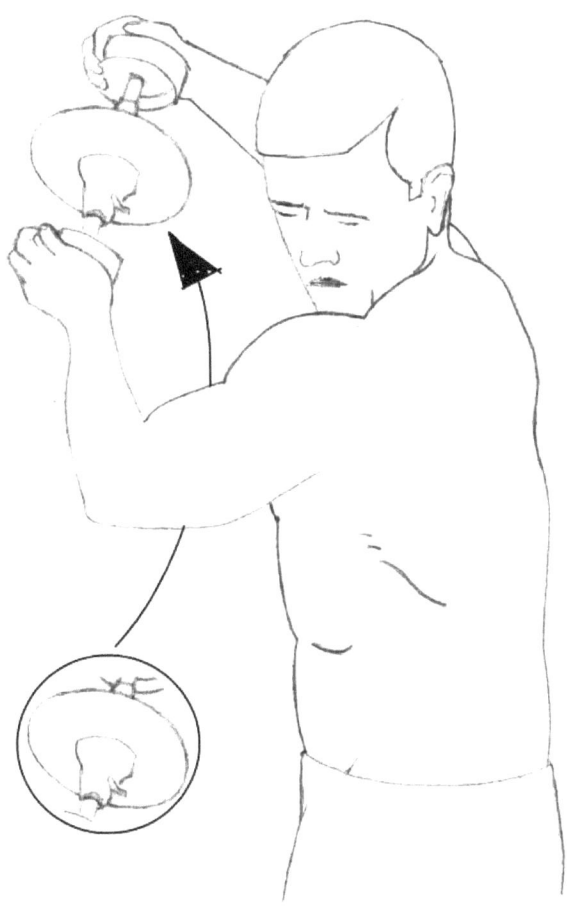

Allow "carry over" trajectory to continue in a flowing parabolic motion, torqueing the lead end of GYROCISOR Power Shuttle to descend.

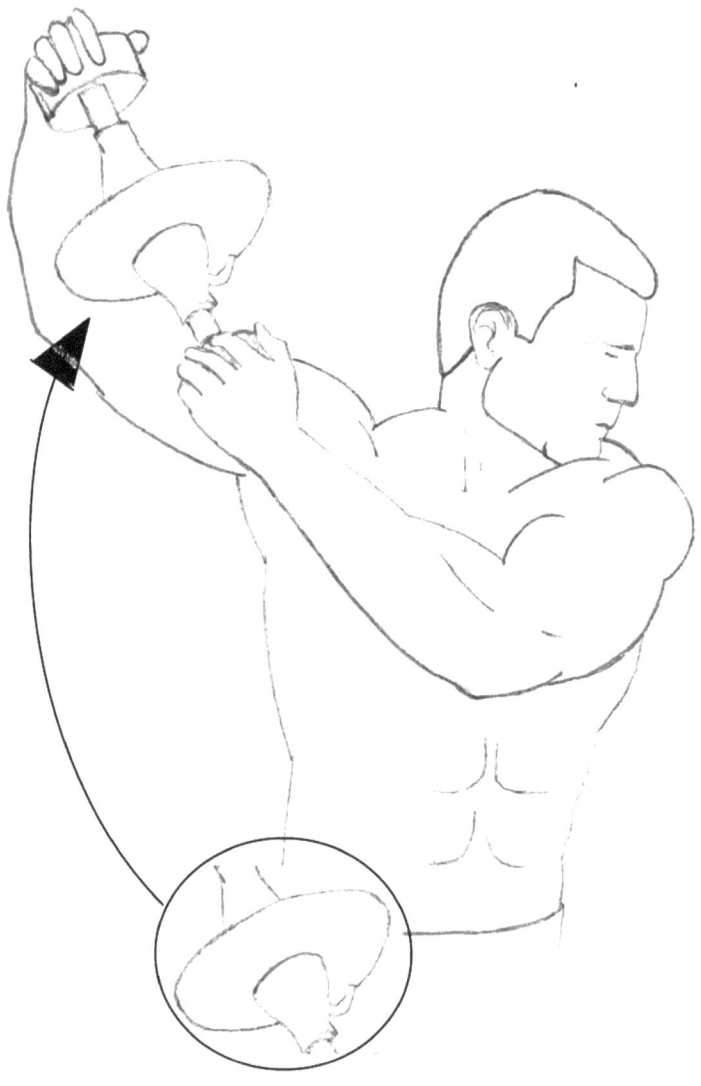

5.) *The Reverse "Torque Tilt"*

Torque the lead end of the descending GYROCISOR Power Shuttle so that it crosses your torso's center of axis.

Allow the Loaded GYROCISOR Power Shuttle to gain angular momentum as it rapidly descends to your left or opposite side.

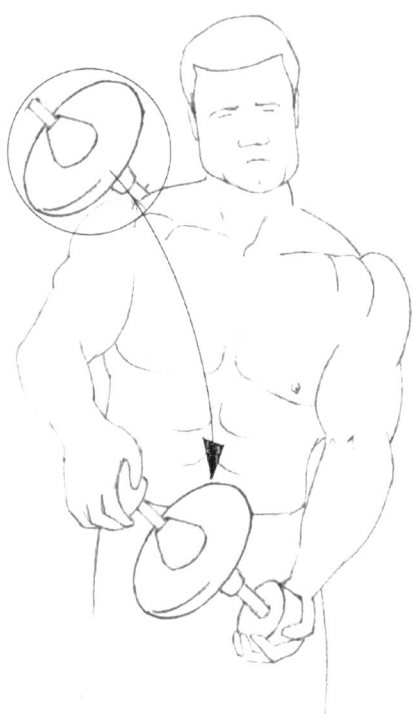

You should begin bending your knees as soon as the GYROCISOR Power Shuttle begins to descend after reaching maximum height.

6.) *The B-Orbital Trajectory*

Use the gained angular momentum to lift the loaded GYROCISOR Power Shuttle above shoulder height in elliptical fashion.

Twist torso and extend bended knees to maximize height of lifted GYROCISOR Power Shuttle.

Allow "carry over" trajectory to continue in a flowing parabolic fashion and let GYROCISOR Power Shuttle descend.

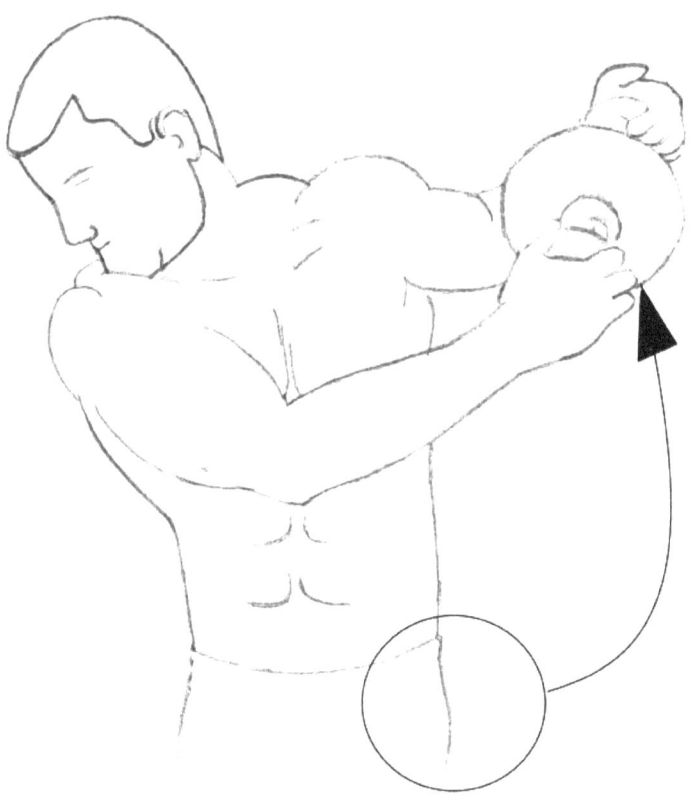

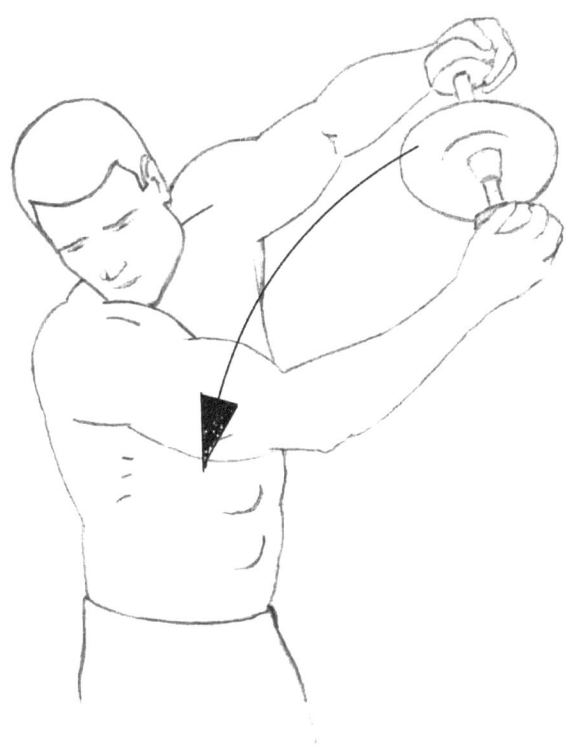

7.) *The Reverse "Torque Tilt"*

Torque the lead end of the descending GYROCISOR Power Shuttle so that it crosses your torso's center of axis.

Allow the Loaded GYROCISOR Power Shuttle to gain angular momentum as it rapidly descends to your right or opposite side.

You should begin bending your knees as soon as the GYROCISOR Power Shuttle begins to descend after reaching maximum height.

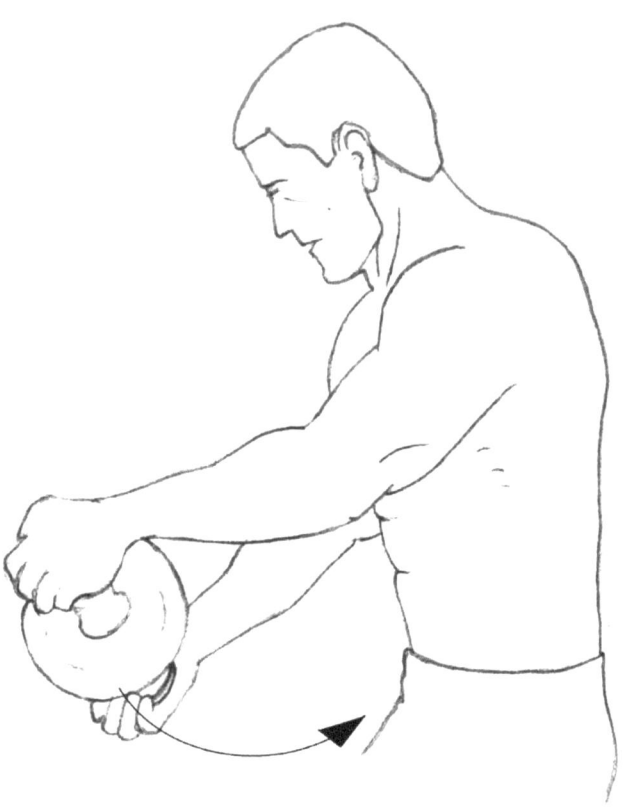

And that's it! To continue the "SuperStroke" maneuver, simply repeat steps 4 - 5 - 6. The loaded and energized GYROCISOR will continue to flow from side to side in a natural simple harmonic fashion because the angular momentum is conserved in the motion.

And it's this "Quantum Dynamic Tension" that you will experience as you are engaged in the GYROCISOR "SuperStroke" maneuver.

The force or kinetic energy of the loaded GYROCISOR Power Shuttle is equal to the force engaging your flexing muscles as you hold on.

So, once you've mastered the GYROCISOR "SuperStroke" maneuver, you'll be on your way to a great cardio and strength workout.

Finally, another way to interpret the "SuperStroke" infinity movement is as a dual trajectory of "Butterfly" wings with the "Quantum Launch" forming the body of the butterfly. One drawback however is that it lacks the appreciation of the dynamic forces at play as the loaded GYROCISOR Power Shuttle traces out the outline of the butterfly wings.

Time Lapse of GYROCISOR "SuperStroke" Maneuver.

The following is a sequence of 14 time lapse photographs demonstrating the basic movements of the GYROCISOR "SuperStroke" maneuver. It begins with the top left photo labeled "1 and continues on a sequential progression to the immediate right and on down.

A.) **#1.) The Power Stance:** This time lapse view demonstrates how to handle the end grips of the GYROCISOR Power Shuttle. Standing upright with legs spread apart over a foot apart to offer a firm, stable stance. Knees should be slightly bent as if about to surf or ski boarding. Arms are extended down with hands firmly gripping each rubber handle.

B.) **#2.) The Quantum Launch:** In this view the user engages the GYROCISOR "SuperStroke" maneuver by lifting the loaded GYROCISOR Power Shuttle, either straight up or in a barbell curling movement. But this upwards motion is halted when the GYROCISOR Power Shuttle reaches chest height.

C.) **#3 & #4.) The Torque Tilt Drop:** This pair of views shows how the leading grip of the GYROCISOR Power Shuttle is tilted in a downward trajectory for a rapid descent to gain the momentum necessary to carrying the GYROCISOR Power Shuttle in an ascending parabolic trajectory. This action commences the first elliptical orbit of the GYROCISOR "SuperStroke" maneuver."

D.) **#5 & #6.) The A-Orbital Trajectory:** Use the gained angular momentum to lift the loaded GYROCISOR Power Shuttle above shoulder height in elliptical fashion. Twist torso and extend bended knees to maximize height of lifted GYROCISOR Power Shuttle.

Allow "carry over" trajectory to continue in a flowing parabolic fashion and let GYROCISOR Power Shuttle descend. The sixth view demonstrates how the descent and final leg of the elliptical orbit.

E.) **#7, #8 & #9.)** The Reverse "Torque Tilt" Drop: These views show how the lead end (bow) of the descending GYROCISOR Power Shuttle is torqued so that it crosses your torso's center of axis. The loaded GYROCISOR Power Shuttle continues to descend toward your left or opposite side.

F.) **#10 & #11.)** The B-Orbital Trajectory: The two views depict the actions of a live GYROCISOR Power Shuttle as its momentum sustains the parabolic trajectory into an elliptical orbit. The apex of this trajectory is determined by the GYRONAUT and should be well within the bounds of safety and injury prevention.

G.) **#12, #13 & #14.)** These three views show the final sequence of one complete repetition of a "SuperStroke" infinity movement. Basically, view #14 is the reverse maneuver of the action depicted in view #4 and essential continues the forward progress of the energized GYROCISOR Power Shuttle into the next elliptical to repeat the routine as if in and endless loop. The final number of orbits to be revolved are to be determined by the practicing GYRONAUT or their physical trainer.

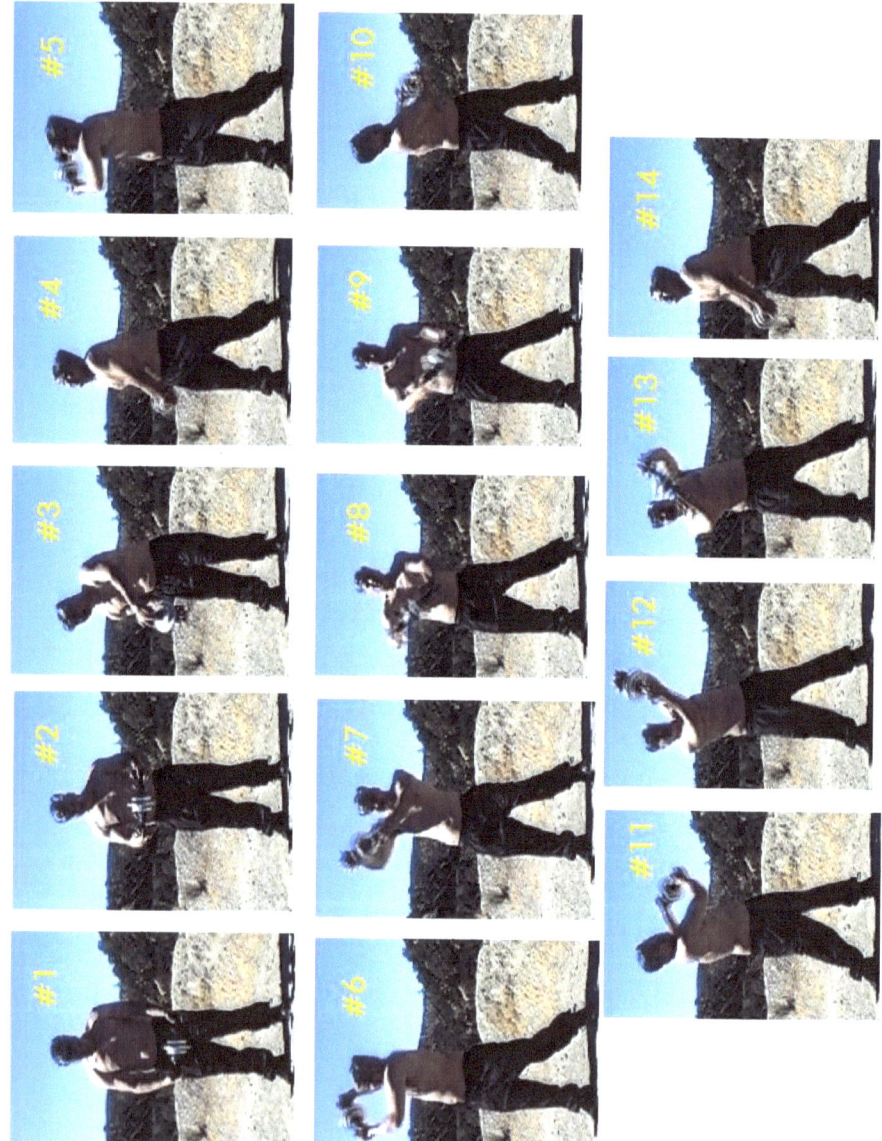

Finally, while an energized or GYROCISOR Power Shuttle must obey the laws of physics, the GYROCISOR "SuperStroke" maneuver is not constrained by the laws governing linear "progressive resistance" exercise routines. Therefore, any twisting of the torso and knee bends can be incorporated in performing the GYROCISOR "SuperStroke" maneuver to enhance the effectiveness of the bi-lateral, dual elliptical orbit.

The other feature of the GYROCISOR Power Shuttle is the ability to quickly and safely add more weight to increase the load. But this is beyond the scope of this chapter and will be addressed within the context of the following chapter.

Chapter Four

How to Build A GYROCISOR Power Shuttle.

The GYROCISOR Power Shuttle is a progressive resistant exercise device that was designed specifically for engaging the GYROCISOR "SuperStroke" maneuver. The sturdy metal construction of the GYROCISOR is purposely intended to support the dynamic G-forces generated by its load during the bi-lateral, dual elliptical trajectory of the "SuperStroke" infinity movement.

The two rubber end handles or grips of the GYROCISOR Power Shuttle provide maximum directional control of the load during the simple harmonic motion (SHM) trajectory. The position of the load or metal plates provides a symmetrical center of gravity that provides easy handling of the energized GYROCISOR Power Shuttle.

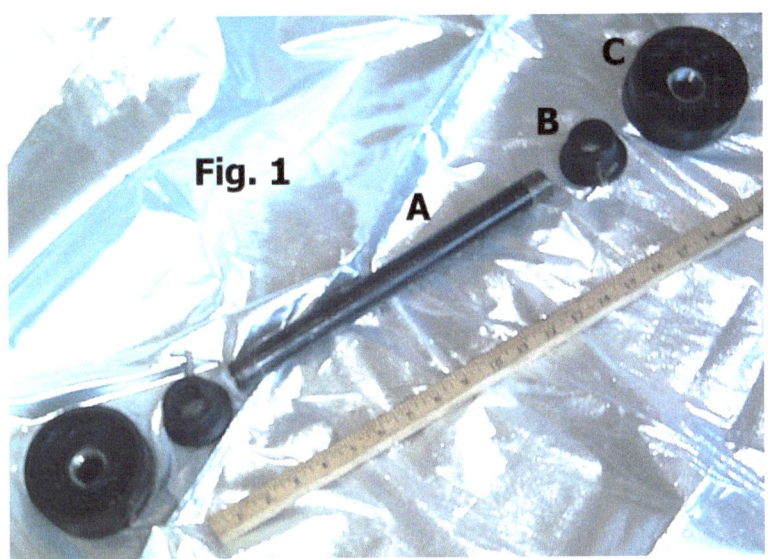

Figure 1 is an exploded view of the GYROCISOR Power Shuttle.

A.) (1) ¾ inch diameter threaded steel pipe; length: 12 inches.

B.) (2) Standard weightlifting collars for dumbbells

C.) (2) Rubber grips measure 4 inches in diameter and 1 ¾ inches deep.

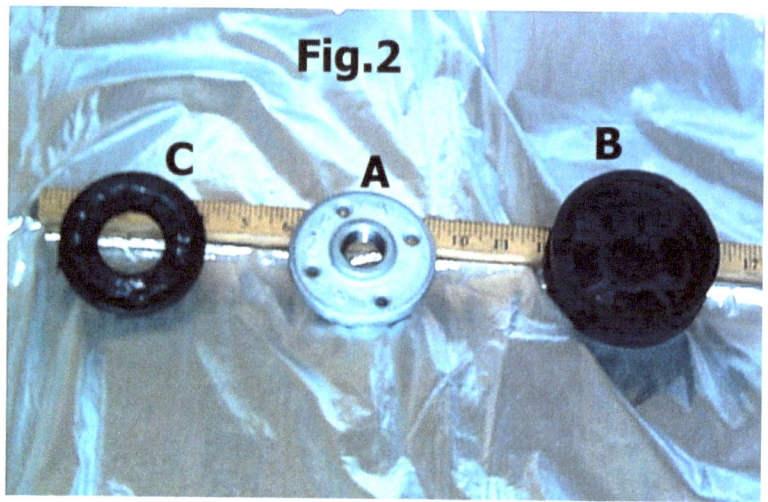

Figure 2 is an exploded view of one rubber grip.

A.) Standard ¾" galvanized floor flange measures 3 ½ inch diameter and weighs 11 ounces.

B.) 3-inch rubber plumber's cap.

C.) Black silicon sealant about ¼ inch thick.

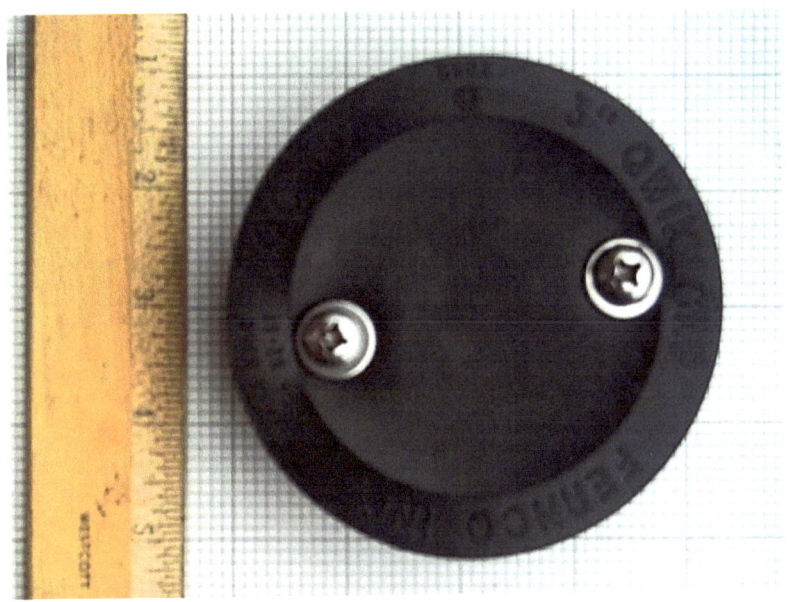

Figure 3 is a view of a Grip complete with two bolts.

Basically, the two rubber (Grips) handles are the only parts that will require assembly.

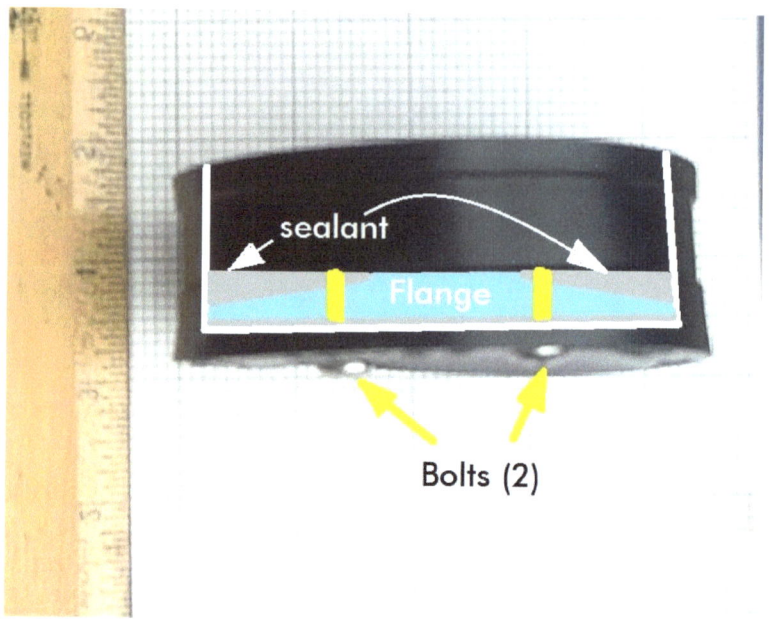

Bolts (2)

How to Assemble a GYROCISOR Power Shuttle Grip.

1.) Insert flange and drill holes for bolts.

2.) Remove flange and prepare the surfaces of flange and interior of rubber cap for sealant.

3.) Apply sealant to inside of rubber cap and insert flange.

4.) Insert each bolt into their respective hole and secure with nut and washer.

5.) Insert pipe or cover center tapered hole. Apply seal to inside of grip. Cover and seal bolts and flange with sealant. Allow sealant to dry or cure for the recommended period before using.

Chapter Five

I Am One with the Universe.

To become one with the universe while engaged in the GYROCISOR "SuperStroke" maneuver with a live and loaded GYROCISOR Power Shuttle means that you and the energized GYROCISOR Power Shuttle are in **sympathetic resonance** or tuned to the **universal harmony** now playing out in the myriad fractal forms of simple harmonic motion (SHM) swinging in dynamic balance between the conservation of angular momentum and the acceleration due to gravity.

While performing the GYROCISOR "SuperStroke" maneuver, the Quantum Dynamic Tension or QDT you experience while holding on to the energized GYROCISOR Power Shuttle centers your whole presence. All your actions are engaged in maintaining that dynamic balance or equilibrium between the counteracting forces of gravity and angular momentum.

As this excerpt from rmcybernetics.com, entitled, "Resonance and Simple Harmonic Motion" explains:

"...Four identical springs are attached to a support. **Each spring has weight with a different mass attached to the end**. If a weight is pulled and released, it will set it in motion bouncing up and down until all its energy is dissipated through friction. As each spring holds a different mass, **they will each have a different fundamental or resonant frequency**. The first spring with the most mass will bounce slowest. We say that this has the lowest resonant frequency out of the four springs. The frequency is simply the number of times the mass bounces up and down each second and is measured in Hertz (Hz).

If the support holding the springs is moved up and down at a set speed, we will see the weights begin to move up and down by different amounts. The amount of displacement of each mass will be dependent upon the frequency that the support is oscillating at.

We will see the maximum displacement when the frequency of the moving support is the same as the resonant frequency of one of the weights. **For example; if the resonant frequency of the first mass and spring is 10Hz then it will move the most when the support is moved up and down at 10Hz. This is known as resonance.** If the support is moving at 9Hz or 11Hz then there will be significantly less movement of the mass. This is because resonance usually occurs when the frequencies match almost exactly.

The exact same principles are used in radios and televisions in order to tune into a specific station. Instead of oscillating springs, it is the electrical currents that are oscillating. By using different components, it is possible to make a circuit that has a resonant frequency that is the same as the radio wave that we wish to detect. At resonance the amplitude of the signal in the circuit will be much higher than any of the other signals which allow us to use just one channel at a time."

Before becoming convoluted beyond reason, let me just clarify by focusing on one key aspect. By emulating the rudimentary motions of the universe with the energized GYROCISOR Power Shuttle, that is, while engaged in the GYROCISOR "SuperStroke" maneuver, we are tapping into that universal dynamism between angular momentum and the acceleration due to gravity.

Gravity is no longer that force we must conquer as if it were a mortal enemy. The force of gravity has become our natural ally. And it is the power we gain from this universal interplay that will allow us to escape the bounds of demeaning exercises and achieve new heights of physical fitness.

We Are Not Robots.

Peering out into the sky at night reveals a dazzling celestial theatre of exploding Supernovas and whirling, twirling galaxies. All intertwined in a timeless gravity dance.

But the amazing thing is, within this universal balance of revolving forces, over the whole expanse of known time, the human physique has evolved to respond and react with the fullest possible range of three dimensional motion. The human body has the ability to perform amazing acrobatic stunts like summersaults and other gymnastic contortions because that's what it was built for.

Basically, we are not robots lacking the smooth articulation of 360-degree flexibility and coordination, that frankly, we just take for granted. We are like the dolphins of the sea or the eagles of the sky, moving with a natural fluidity that translates into absolute mastery of the immediate macro environment.

With our minds and bodies fully wired for 360-degree range of motion, the GYROCISOR "SuperStroke" maneuver allows us to mimic the manner by which the universe operates. This induces a synergy of mind and body that effectively opens a door to our universal soul.

Yes, this is not your typical grunt and strain exercise. Of course it is strenuous by nature, but it is a transcendent exertion in that it tunes your will to the eternal will of the Universe.

Why is this relevant to your life? Well, for one thing, stress or those external forces, real or imagined, which trigger our visceral reactions of fight or flight, are basically dumping powerful chemical substances into the blood stream. Of course, for an epoch of time in the survival of man, this boost was a definite life saver.

Unfortunately, most of these modern day stresses cannot be resolved either by a fight or flight response. So, day after day, these minute chemical doses are not consumed in actual physical exertion. Instead the traces begin to accumulate causing a chronic chemical imbalance that persistently acts to disturb or upset the body's natural homeostasis responses.

Another way to consider these reactions is that stress is an external collision that puts a negative spin on our healthy, positive energy. That's why physical activities like walking or running are superbly effective in neutralizing or "working out" the chemical imbalances.

And would it not stand to reason that the sooner these stress-induced chemical imbalances were effective neutralized, the better. After all, it's these chemical imbalances that are so disruptive to the body's natural homeostasis balance and not the imagined recollection of the stressful encounter.

This is why the GYROCISOR "SuperStroke" maneuver can be highly effective as an exercise. Anywhere or anytime someone is confronted by a negative stress inducer; they can use the GYROCISOR Power Shuttle the chemical imbalances back into equilibrium.

It's similar to picking up a sledgehammer every time something aggravates your senses and whacking the crap out of something. Because with a loaded GYROCISOR Power Shuttle and the GYROCISOR "SuperStroke" maneuver you can literally go berserk. But when you're done letting it all go, you'll just feel excellent and nothing has been destroyed.

And because no one gets hurt and no furniture or glassware damaged, it truly is all good. In effect, by channeling those hostilities and aggressions into the GYROCISOR exercise, you'll have spun that negative agitation into a positive flow.

And so by becoming one with the universe, the force will be with you.

www.ingramcontent.com/pod-product-compliance
Lightning Source LLC
Chambersburg PA
CBHW040746010626
45792CB00027B/300